An Evidence-Based approach to Frontline & Middle-Level Managers Handoff

A PRACTICAL TOOL FOR LEADERSHIP HANDOFF: LSBAR

CLINICAL DECISION SUPPORT (CDSS)

ENVIRONMENT OF CARE (EOC)

HUMAN RESOURCES MANAGEMENT (HRM)

Author: Rudolph George Newman, DNP

Leadership

Situation

Background

Assessment

Recommendation

About the Author

Dr. Rudolph G. Newman is a two-time graduate of Walden University where he completed his Doctor of Nursing Practice (DNP) in 2016 and Master of Science in Nursing Leadership and Management in 2009. Dr. Newman, a Jamaica native, began his journey shortly after high school by obtaining an Associate's degree in Agricultural Science from the College of Agriculture in Jamaica in 1989. Within that same year, he joined the United States Army as a PFC and completed Basic Training at Fort Jackson, South Carolina.

Dr. Newman started his military career as a Power Generation Mechanic and was assigned to the 156th Maintenance Company in Nuremberg, Germany and deployed to Desert Shield/Desert Storm from 1991-1992. After this brief deployment, he was stationed with the 194th Armor Brigade at Fort Knox, Kentucky where he earned both Soldier of the Month and Soldier of the Quarter awards and entered the Noncommissioned Officer's rank of sergeant. Dr. Newman decided to further his education while in the military and completed the Practical Nurse Course with Phase II at Fort Gordon GA in 1994. During his military career, he completed many leadership training up to the rank of rank of Sergeant First Class.

While serving in the Army, Dr. Newman received several awards and decorations. His awards include the Army Commendation Medal 3rd Award, Army Good Conduct Medal 2nd Award, NCO development Ribbon w/ Numeral 12, Army Commendation Medal 1st Award, Army Good Conduct Medal 1st Award, National Service Medal, Southwest Asia Service Medal, Kuwait Liberation Medal (KU), Kuwait Liberation Medal (SA), Army Achievement Medal, and the Army Service Ribbon.

Publication: Frontline and Middle-Level Nursing Leader Transition Within the Military Health System ©

After his military career, he began working as an LPN contract Critical Care Nurse. During his ICU stay, Dr. Newman received his Associates of Science Nursing degree at Augusta University. He later became a certified Critical Care Registered Nurse (CCRN). Dr. Newman is the recipient of numerous civilian awards and recognitions to include Nursing Excellence Award 2014, Nurse Researcher of the Year Award (CSRA) 2014, Nursing Excellence Award 2011, Reflection of Nursing Spirit Award 2011, and the Civilian Achievement Medal 2010.

Dr. Newman's expertise evolved through multiple lines of efforts where he has served as a soldier leader, staff nurse, Adjunct Clinical Instructor, Nursing Supervisor, Program Developer, and his latest role as the Director of a Clinical Nurse Transition Program. He is also a TeamSTEPPS Master Trainer, Mock Code Coordinator, Affiliation Agreement Coordinator for Nursing, Nurse Summer Training Program Coordinator, and Instructor for multiple courses to include evidence-based practice.

Introduction

The landscape of healthcare delivery is changing rapidly. Thus, requires a multifaceted approach to achieving the desired outcomes of safe, effective, patient-centered, timely, efficient, and equitable health care. The prospect of maintaining a cycle of continuous process improvements within the clinical setting hinges on frontline leaders and middle-level managers, who are prepared to execute the mission, motivate, supervise, coach, and mentor their staff. Many compounding factors such as the lack of a proper handoff mechanism, role orientation, and constant mission changes leave the newly assigned frontline leaders and middle-level managers unprepared to meet the clinical, administrative, and human resources demands of the position.

As a nurse leader, it is my sincere hope that you will maximize your time and talent using this handy guide. In many cases, you know what to do, but are without the tools to get the job done efficiently. Taking over a new department is stressful enough coupled with the fact that your predecessor is most likely not available or accessible to you. The tool provided here will help you collect the information that you need to get started on a successful leadership journey.

Publication: Frontline and Middle-Level Nursing Leader Transition Within the Military Health System ©

Why You Need a Handoff

1. You are new to the position

2. You are new to the organization

3. You cannot possibly know everything about the new position

4. The last position you had was nothing like the new one

5. Your staff is awaiting your decision

6. Your leaders are awaiting your reports

10. Patient safety is your number one concern

11. Staff satisfaction depends on your leadership

12. You need a baseline

13. Continuity of care

14. This is your first leadership/manager role

15. Do you know what works and what does not?

16. What you need to know and what can wait

17. Where are your support systems?

18. Opportunity to ask questions

19. Opportunity for verification

20. An opportunity to review any relevant data

"Ineffective hand-off communication is recognized as a critical patient safety problem in health care; in fact, an estimated 80% of serious medical errors involve miscommunication between caregivers during the transfer of patients." TJC, 2012).

Publication: Frontline and Middle-Level Nursing Leader Transition Within the Military Health System ©

Simplifying the Complex Relationships within the Practice Setting

Figure 1. Concept Diagram

Transformational Leadership Induction Program (TLIP) module

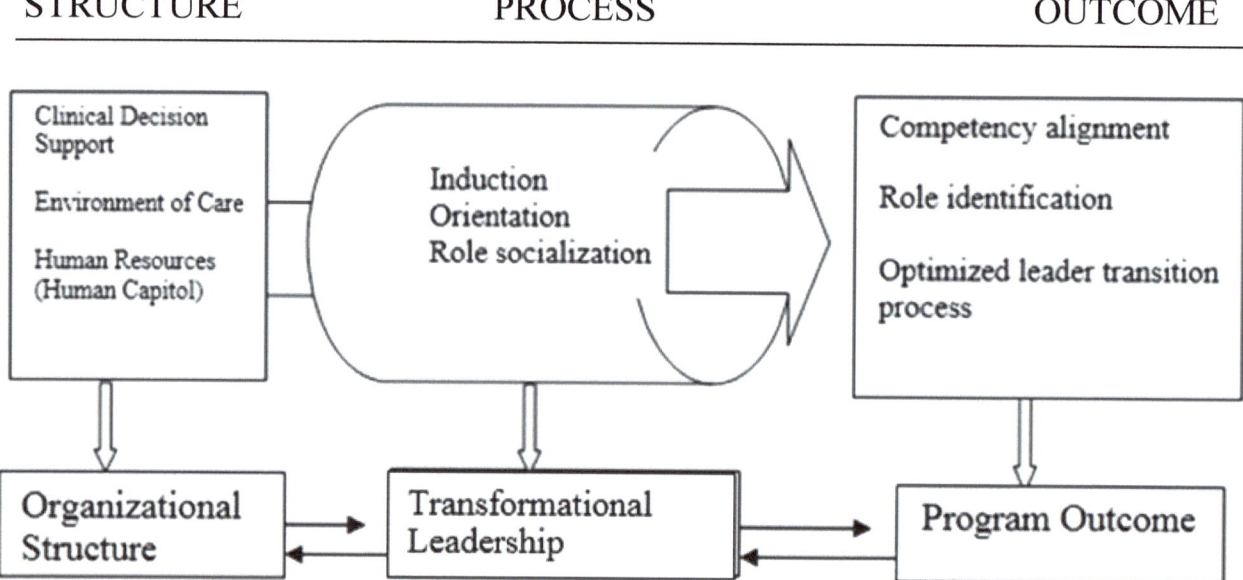

Frontline leaders and middle-level managers are responsible for promoting and establishing practice environments that balance complex demands and perspectives (Laschinger & Wong, 2010). The CDSS comprises the information technology infrastructure that supports evidence-based decision-making through data management. Primarily, the CDSS facilitates the provision of care in complex work environments through point of care testing, alerts and reminders, treatment order set, and real-time information for clinicians to engage in patient care decisions (HealthIT.gov. 2013).

The environment of care process includes The Joint Commission's (TJC) standard requirements for safety, security, hazards and material waste, fire safety, medical equipment and utilities (Mills, 2013). Understanding the roles and responsibilities of the position include the environment of care systems processes, policies, and procedures critical to the unit/organizational outcomes. The third overarching component of the conceptual TLIP model (Figure 1) encompasses human resources (HRM) and human capital management (HCM). The policies and practices of governing people management include scheduling, multiple types of leave policies, equal opportunity and equal employment opportunity, workers compensation, Labor Union rules and practices, hiring practices, disciplinary practices, pay and compensation, conflict management, performance evaluation, promotions, and much more.

Leadership SBAR Matrix in (Figure 2) outlined the handoff process that represents the transfer of responsibility and accountability from one person to the next in a clear format while allowing the receiver to acknowledge the information and ask questions for clarity (AHRQ, 2014). The Status, Team, Environment, and Progress (STEP) are embedded within the diagram to represent an assessment of the background information the transitioning leader needs to know. The guiding philosophy to frame the assessment in TeamSTEPPS is to reduce the stress of introducing new tools that might cause confusion.

6

The Aim: Bridge the Transition GAP

Figure 3

- Bridge the transition gap
- Facilitate role orientation, induction, and socialization

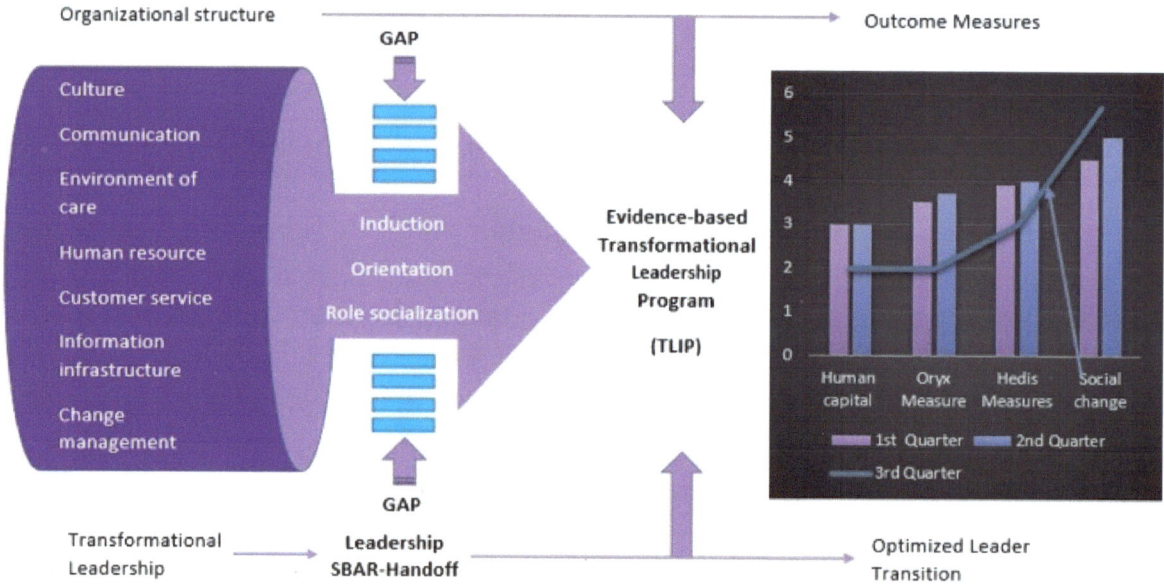

The future of healthcare relies in part on leaders that are transformational in their thinking and actions. According to Caillier (2014), there are some significant characteristics of transformational leadership:

- leaders emphasis on the collective vision

- inspirational motivation

- individual consideration

- intellectual stimulation

Today's leader must confront generational differences and leverage technology in their quest to achieve positive staff and customer experiences and outcomes. Consequently, the gap (Figure 3) between current leaders and the new millennial workforce requires an evidenced-based approach that encompasses aligning traditional barriers to create a bridge of opportunity to preserve quality, advance progress, reduce cost, and generate interest in the nursing professional development.

Figure 4.

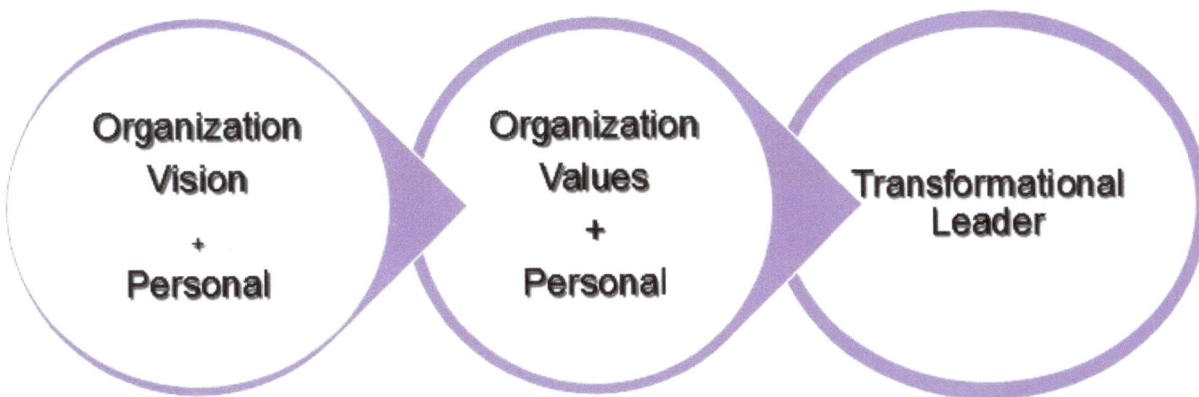

In traditional of nursing practice, there are multiple avenues and pathways to the upper rung of the leadership ladder. However, as Watts (2013) suggested, the transformational leader needs to align his/her aspirations with the values and attributes of the organization's vision and mission (Figure 4). Inarguably, the next generation of nurse leaders must be in tune with the speed of change in technology, the work ethic of the next generation, and the evolving demands of their clientele.

My goal is that you will find this handoff tool practical and applicable to your situation. At the bedside, there is no doubt that a standardized handoff practice mitigates errors in practice. On the side of leadership, it is less likely for handoff to occur. The reality is that as the nurse leader, you have to lead. Having a tool and a stubby pencil might be your best chance of taking the job head-on.

Matrix

Figure 2. Leadership SBAR

Matrix

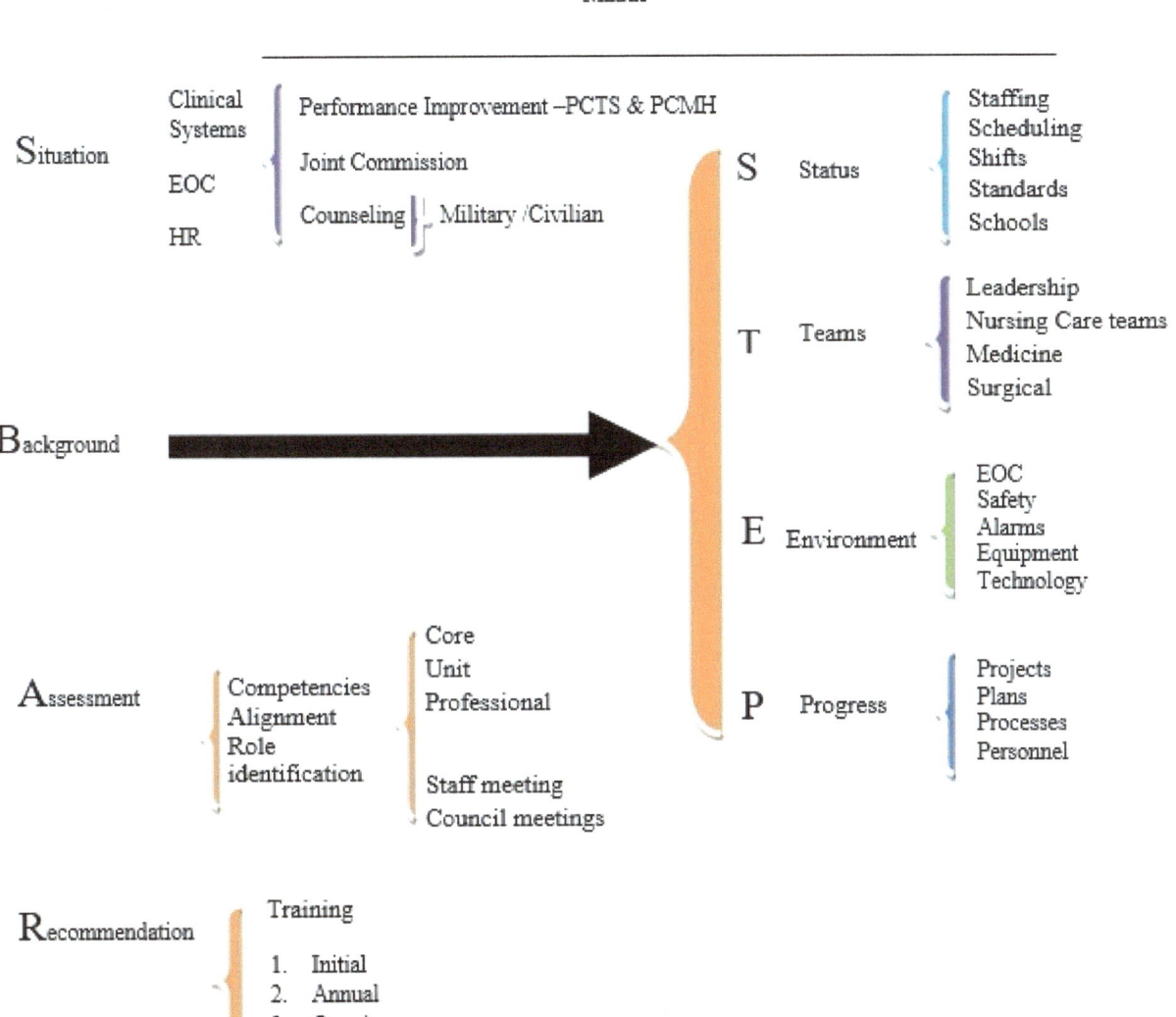

JC-Joint commission   EOC-environment of care

PCTS-Patient CaringTouch System   PCMH-Patient Centered Medical Home

HR-Human Resources

About Your UNIT/CLINIC/SECTION STRUCTURE

Unit Type: Select all that applies to your situation

☐ Critical Care	☐ OR	☐ Troop Medical Clinic
☐ Med/Surg	☐ GYN	☐ Out Patient Clinic
☐ Progressive Care	☐ GI	☐ Ortho
☐ Telemetry	☐ GU	☐ Other
☐ PSYCH	☐ EENT	☐ Ed & Trng
☐ ER	☐ RTF	

Patient /Client Population

☐ Active Duty	☐ Adults	☐ Other
☐ Civilian	☐ Pediatric	
☐ Contractors	☐ Beneficiary	

Unit Size

#of Beds _____ #of Female beds _____ #of Male beds _____ #of Pediatrics_____

Psychiatric Beds _____ Recovery Beds_____ N/A_____

Number of Personnel

Physician_____PA_____APRN_____RN_____RN_____LPN_____CNA_____TECH_____

MSA _____Secretary _____Other _____

Full Time Staff_____ Part Time Staff_____ Contract Staff_____

Barrowed Staff_____ Transient Staff_____ Volunteer Staff _____

Publication: Frontline and Middle-Level Nursing Leader Transition Within the Military Health System ©

NOTES: What other services does your unit /clinic/section provide?

_____

_____

_____

_____

_____

_____

_____

_____

_____

_____

_____

_____

_____

_____

_____

_____

_____

_____

_____

_____

_____

_____

_____

_____

_____

_____

_____

Publication: Frontline and Middle-Level Nursing Leader Transition Within the Military Health System ©

Start Your New Role with Knowledge

Quick Notes

_____
_____
_____
_____
_____
_____

Quick Notes

_____
_____
_____
_____
_____
_____

Quick Notes

_____
_____
_____
_____
_____
_____

Situation

Clinical Decisional Support Systems

Environment of Care (EOC)

Human Resource Management (HRM)

Management is doing things right; leadership is doing the right things.

(Peter F. Drucker, 2001)

Clinical Decision Support Systems

Enterprise Contact #:		
Identify the clinical decision systems within the work setting		
System Name/ Type	Purpose	Local Contacts Name/Phone /Email

Publication: Frontline and Middle-Level Nursing Leader Transition Within the Military Health System ©

Notes Page: Are there any expected changes or new systems on the horizon?

_____

_____

_____

_____

_____

_____

_____

_____

_____

_____

_____

_____

_____

_____

_____

_____

_____

_____

_____

_____

_____

Environment of Care

<table>
<tr><td colspan="5"></td></tr>
<tr><td colspan="5">If deficiencies are found, document the date that work order was placed and recorded into work order log.</td></tr>
<tr><td rowspan="2">The Joint Commission</td><td>Last visit</td><td>Outcomes</td><td>Areas needing improvement</td><td>Recommendation</td></tr>
<tr><td></td><td></td><td></td><td></td></tr>
<tr><td rowspan="6">Unit Performance Improvement Projects</td><td>Title</td><td>Start Date</td><td>Status</td><td>Comments</td></tr>
<tr><td></td><td></td><td></td><td></td></tr>
<tr><td></td><td></td><td></td><td></td></tr>
<tr><td></td><td></td><td></td><td></td></tr>
<tr><td></td><td></td><td></td><td></td></tr>
<tr><td></td><td></td><td></td><td></td></tr>
</table>

Publication: Frontline and Middle-Level Nursing Leader Transition Within the Military Health System ©

Care Delivery Models	Patient Centered Care Model (Inpatient setting)			
	_____			
	_____			
	_____			
	_____			
	_____			
	Patient Centered Care Model (Outpatient setting)			
	_____			
	_____			
	_____			
	_____			
	Other			
	_____			
	_____			
	_____			
	_____			

	Unit Practice Council	Nurse Practice Council	Leadership Practice Council	Nurse Executive Council
Status				
Contacts				

Safety Concerns

Work Orders	
Work order #	Status:
Work order #	Status:
Work order #	Status:

17

Publication: Frontline and Middle-Level Nursing Leader Transition Within the Military Health System ©

Human Resources Management

Military Personnel	Grade/Rank	Evaluation Due	Counseling	Records Complete	Disciplinary Action	Promotions
Comments						

Gains and Loss	
Detailed	
Leave	
Medical	
Pass	
Retirement	
Schools	

Notes

_____

_____

_____

_____

_____

Publication: Frontline and Middle-Level Nursing Leader Transition Within the Military Health System ©

Civilian Personnel	Position types (RN, LPN etc.)	Evaluation Due	Counseling	Records Complete	Disciplinary Actions	Awards
Comments						

Gains and Loss	
Detailed	
Leave	
Medical	
Pass	
Retirement	
Transfer	
Schools	

Hiring Actions						
Staff Type	Area of need	#of vacancies	Date action initiated	Target date	Status	HR Contact

19

Notes Page: Note areas that need immediate attention.

_____

_____

_____

_____

_____

_____

_____

_____

_____

_____

_____

_____

_____

_____

_____

_____

_____

_____

Quick Notes

_____
_____
_____
_____

_____
_____Quick
Notes

_____
_____
_____
_____
_____

_____
_____Quick
Notes

_____
_____
_____
_____
_____
_____
_____
_____
_____
_____
_____

Quick Notes

_____
_____
_____
_____
_____
_____
_____
_____
_____
_____
_____

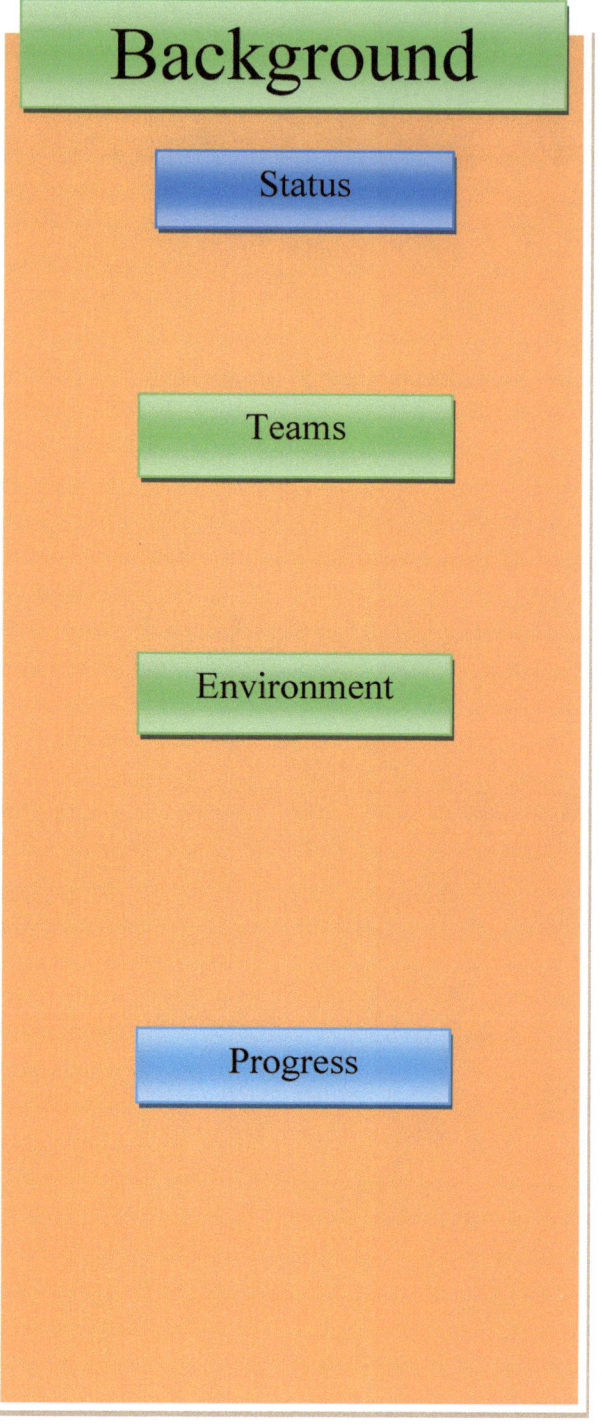

"Psychology keeps trying to vindicate human nature. History keeps undermining the effort."
(MASON COOLEY, City Aphorisms)

21

Status

Items	Questions	Notes
Staffing	• Who makes the schedules?	Obtain a copy of the TDA/staffing document
	• What are your responsibilities for scheduling?	
	• What is the staffing mix?	What is the staffing methodology?
Scheduling	• Self-scheduling	
	• What are the scheduling rules?	

	• Leave and Pass rule?
	  • Convalescent leave
	  • Sick leave
	  • Annual leave
	  • Leave without pay
	  • Absent without leave
	  • Military leave
		What works/flex scheduling

Shifts	• Rotating shifts • Days • Evenings • Nights • On call • Cross covering • Straight 8s	**Ask about workflow**

Publication: Frontline and Middle-Level Nursing Leader Transition Within the Military Health System ©

Standards	• TeamSTEPPS • Metric and Dashboards • Medical Command Polices • Hospital Policies • Nursing Policies • Evidence-based Practice	**Where are the policies located?**
Schools/Training	• Military Education • Civilian Education • Staff Education • Unit Education	**Criteria/contracts/status reports**

Teams

		Notes
Leadership		
Nursing Care Teams		
Medicine		
Surgical		
Performance Improvement		
Hazmat		

Notes

Environment

		Notes
	Patient Care Environment	
Safety	<ul><li>Fire/Electrical Safety</li><li>Medication Safety</li><li>Fall Prevention</li><li>Code Blue</li><li>Infection Control</li><li>Clinical Alarms</li><li>Code system</li></ul>	
Equipment	<ul><li>Beds Management</li><li>Key Control</li><li>Hand Receipt</li></ul>	
Items Turn-in	Status	
Purchase	Status	
Damage Items	Status	
Technology	Wireless Devices	
other		

Progress

	Notes		
Projects	• Unit Projects		
	• Section Projects		
	• Hospital projects		

	Unit Training Plans	Monthly	Quarterly	Annual
Plans	• Mock Code			
	• Evacuation			
	• Preceptor Course			
	• Charge Nurse Course			
	• SHARP			
	•			
	• TeamSTEPPS			
	• Customer Service			

Processes	• Leave and Passes	
	• Temporary duty assignment	
	• Patient Safety Reports	
	• Evaluations	
	• Performance Improvement	
	• FOCUS-PDCA	
	• DMAIC	
	• EBP	
	• Research	
	•	

Personnel	• Performance improvement	
	Rating Schemes	
	Military	
	Civilian	
	Competency Validation	
	CBO	
	Initial	
	Ongoing	

NOTES

_____

_____

_____

_____

_____

_____

_____

_____

Publication: Frontline and Middle-Level Nursing Leader Transition Within the Military Health System ©

What do you need to move **forward?**

Quick notes

_____
_____
_____
_____
_____
_____
_____
_____

Quick notes

_____
_____
_____
_____
_____
_____
_____
_____

Quick notes

_____
_____
_____
_____
_____
_____
_____

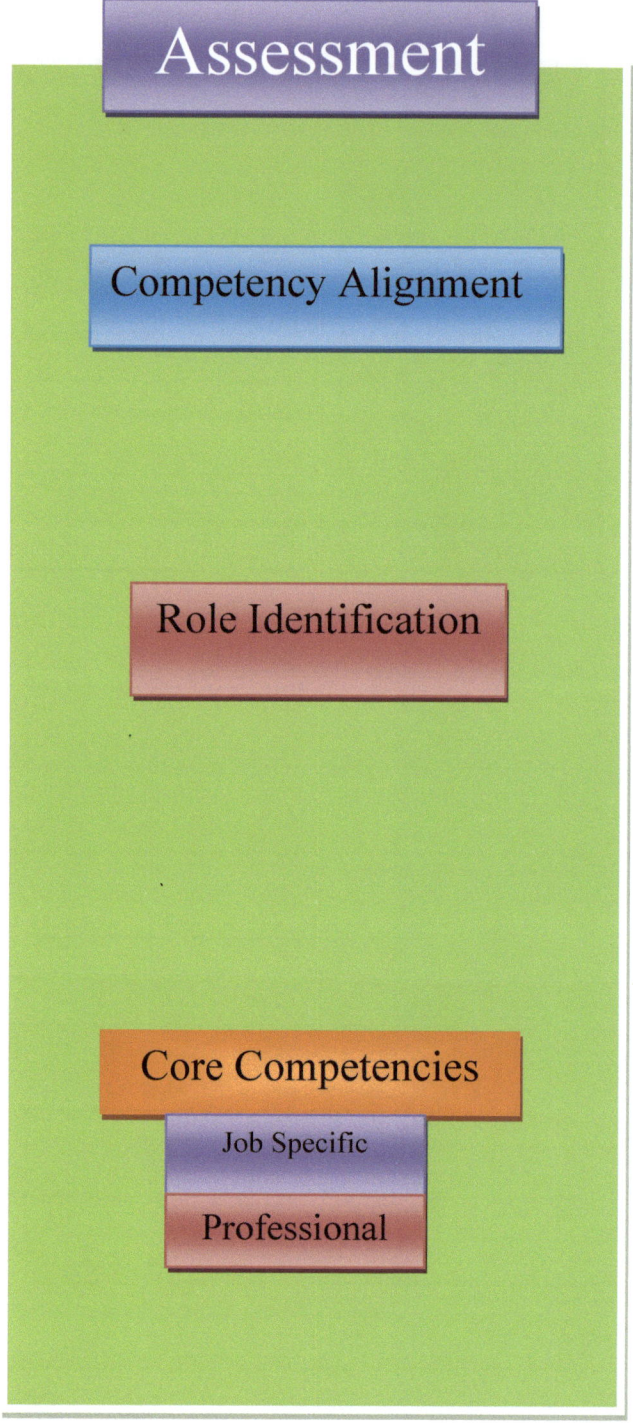

The highs of great men reached and kept were not attained by sudden flight, but they while their companions slept, were toiling upwards through the night

Poet Henry Wadsworth Longfellow

Publication: Frontline and Middle-Level Nursing Leader Transition Within the Military Health System ©

Competency Alignment

Complete Leadership Initial Competency Based Orientation (CBO)

Complete Nurse Manager Skills Inventory (AONE)

Role Identification

	Who	When	Where
Assistant Nurse Manager			
Leadership Practice Council			
Nurse Executive Council			
Committees			

Publication: Frontline and Middle-Level Nursing Leader Transition Within the Military Health System ©

Core Competencies

- Job Specific & Professional

Leading the Unit/Section/Clinic:

- Change Management

- Problems solving and decision-making

- Managing politics and influencing others

- Risks Management

- Setting vision and strategy

- Workload management

- Budget and finance knowledge and skills

- Organizational Knowledge

Leading self:

- Demonstrate core values

- Lead by example

- Self-management

- Emotional intelligence

Publication: Frontline and Middle-Level Nursing Leader Transition Within the Military Health System ©

- Communicate effectively

- Develop others

- Value diversity and difference

- Build and maintain relationships

- Manage teams and work groups

Society for Human Resources Management, 2008)

Notes

_____
_____
_____
_____
_____
_____
_____
_____
_____
_____
_____
_____
_____
_____
_____
_____
_____
_____

Publication: Frontline and Middle-Level Nursing Leader Transition Within the Military Health System ©

Recommendations

What are your recommendations to move forward?

Quick Notes

_____
_____
_____
_____
_____
_____
_____
_____

Quick Notes

_____
_____
_____
_____
_____
_____
_____

Quick Notes

_____
_____
_____
_____
_____
_____
_____

Recommendations

Training needs assessment

Initial –Strengths, Weakness Opportunity & Threats

Annual-process reviews and feedback assessments Ongoing-staff recognition & feedback

Publication: Frontline and Middle-Level Nursing Leader Transition Within the Military Health System ©

In the absence of an incumbent, develop an action plan based on your assessment.

Strategies could include:

- Staff survey

- Conduct a SWOT

- Seek out a mentor

- Review regulations

- Do not make any immediate change unless necessary

- Conduct a needs assessment

- Collaborate with colleagues from other departments

Notes

_____

_____

_____

_____

_____

_____

_____

_____

Publication: Frontline and Middle-Level Nursing Leader Transition Within the Military Health System ©

Turnover

Turnover affects an organization in multiple ways. Knudson (2014) noted, "Loss of revenue, decreased employee satisfaction, increased operational inefficiencies, and substantial monetary loss associated with the high costs of recruiting and onboarding processes"(p. 1). Ineffective leadership handoff or the lack thereof creates opportunities for unfavorable outcomes. The absence of programs or handoff processes to assist the newly assigned frontline leaders and middle-level managers in the transition to their roles and functions is inconsistent with the patient safety culture.

The prospect of maintaining a cycle of continuous process improvements within the clinical setting hinges on frontline leaders and middle-level managers, who are prepared to execute the mission, motivate, supervise, coach, and mentor the staff. According to White and Dudley-Brown (2012), "Leaders help organizations cope with change" (p. 94). The clinical leadership challenge that currently exists is a revolving door where frontline leaders and middle managers frequently transition in and out of leadership and management positions without receiving a handoff.

Handoff or Handover

The process of handoff or handover has been recognized as a patient safety concern at the bedside between oncoming and off going shifts (Wakefeild, Ragan, Brandt, & Tregnago, 2012). According to Gordon and Findley (2011), the process ensured accurate and reliable communication transfer between the involved parties. However, the same emphasis is not given to frontline leaders and middle-level managers. Dewey (2012) noted, "People are naturally anxious about transition and what it means for their particular job or role. Transitional environments are rife with questions, uncertainty, and fear of the unknown" (p. 136). Similarly,

33

the staff bears some of the anxiety, as they too want to know how the leadership change will affect them (Dewey, 2012). Dragoni, Park, Soltis, and Forte-Trammell (2014) identified several elements critical to frontline leader development to include role knowledge, figuring out boundaries, and the need for a supervisor to model effective leadership behaviors.

According to The Joint Commission (2012, p.1), "Ineffective hand-off communication is recognized as a critical patient safety problem in health care; in fact, an estimated 80% of serious medical errors involve miscommunication between caregivers during the transfer of patients." An effective handoff is deliberate in its intent and purpose to communicate information between sender and receiver (TJC, 2012). A plethora of literature is accessible that addresses nurse handoff between caregivers. However, the literature is less robust with respect to the handoff at the nurse manager level.

The role of leadership in patient safety extends beyond their HRM duties to encompass the guardian of the culture of safety (Sammer & James, 2011). Without proper handoff between incumbents and successors, these nurse leaders are faced with the difficult task of leading with uncertainty through trial and error. Bridging the transition gap through the deliberate transfer of responsibility using a standardized handoff process is an initial step towards building and sustaining high-reliability within the organization (Chassin & Loeb, 2014).

Handoff Tools and Strategies

In a systematic review of the literature on handoff mnemonics, Riesenberg, Leitzsch, and Little (2009) reviewed 46 articles and identified 24 mnemonic addressing handoffs. The most frequently used mnemonic (69.6%) published over a three years period was the SBAR (Situation, Background, Assessment, and Recommendation) tool (Riesenberg et al., 2009). The use of SBAR as a handoff tool is clearly documented in the literature and has been used to pass patient care information from nurse to nurse, physician to physician, and among interdisciplinary teams (Boaro et al., 2010; Cornell, Townsend, Gervis, Yates, & Vardaman, 2014).

According to the Institute for Health Improvement (2015), SBAR was developed by Michael Leonard, MD, and colleagues at Kaiser Permanente in Colorado. Following the landmark IOM (1999) report *"To Err is Human,"* "The Agency for Healthcare Research and Quality (AHRQ) in conjunction with the Department of Defense released Teams Tools and Strategies to Enhance Performance and Patent Safety (TeamSTEPPS) as the national standard for team training in healthcare" (King et al., n.d., p. 4). The SBAR handoff tool was published as one of the communication instruments in TeamSTEPPS training.

Resources

Agency for Healthcare Research and Quality. (2015). *TeamSTEPPS 2.0.* Retrieved from http://www.ahrq.gov/professionals/education/curriculumtools/ TEAMSTEPPS/instructor/index.html

Agency for Healthcare Research and Quality (2014). *TeamSTEPPS 2.0: Core curriculum.* Retrieved from http://www.ahrq.gov/professionals/education/curriculumtools/ TEAMSTEPPS/instructor/index.html

Ali, N., Jan, S., Ali, A., &Tariq, M. (2014). Transformational and transactional leadership as predictors of job satisfaction, commitment, perceived performance and turnover intention. *Life Science Journal, 11*(5s), 48-53.

Boaro, N., Fancott, C., Baker, R., Velji, K., &Andreoli, A. (2010). Using SBAR to improve communication in interprofessional rehabilitation teams. Situation-Background-Assessment-Recommendation. Journal of Interprofessional Care, 24(1), 111-114. doi:10.3109/13561820902881601.

Caillier, J. (2014). Toward a better understanding of the relationship between transformational leadership, public service motivation, mission valence, and employee performance: A study. *Public Personnel Management, 43*(2), 218-239. doi:10.1177/0091026014528478.

Chassin, M. R.,& Loeb, J, M. (2013). High-reliability health Care: Getting there from here. Milbank Quarterly, 91(3), 459-490. doi: 10.1111/1468-0009.12023.

Dewey, B. I. (2012). In transition: The special nature of leadership change. Journal of Library Administration, 52(1), 133-144. doi:10.1080/01930826.2012.629965

Dragoni, L., Park, H., Soltis, J., & Forte-Trammell, S. (2014). Show and tell: How supervisors facilitate leader development among transitioning leaders. Journal of Applied Psychology. 99(1), 66–86. doi: 10.1037/a0034452.

Gordon, M., & Findley, R. (2011). Educational interventions to improve handover in health care: A systematic review. *Medical Education, 45*(11), 1081-1089. doi:10.1111/j.1365-2923.2011.04049.x

HealthIT.gov. (2013). *Clinical decision support (CDS).* Retrieved from http://www.healthit.gov/policy-researchers-implementers/clinical-decisionsupport-cds

Institute of Medicine, Committee on Quality of Health Care in America. (2001). *Crossing the quality chasm: A new health system for the 21ˢᵗ century.*Washington, DC: National Academy Press.

King, H. B., Battles, J., Baker, D. P., Alonso, A., Salas, E., Webster, J., &…,(does this means more names not included?) Salisbury, M. (n.d.). TeamSTEPPS™: Team strategies and tools to enhance performance and patient safety.

Knudson, L. (2014). Developing internal talent necessary to fill perioperative leadership roles. *ARON Connections. 99*(2), 1-10. doi.org/10.1016/S0001-2092 (13)01401-4

Pearson, A., Laschinger, H., Porritt, K., Jordan, Z., Tucker, D., & Long, L. (2007). Comprehensive systematic review of evidence on developing and sustaining nursing leadership that fosters a healthy work environment in healthcare. *JBI Library of Systematic Reviews. 5*(5):279-343.

Riesenberg, L. A., Leitzsch, J., & Little, B. W. (2009). Systematic review of handoff mnemonics literature. American Journal of Medical Quality, 24(3), 196-204. doi: 10.1177/1062860609332512.

Sammer, C. E., & James, B. R. (2011). Patient safety culture: The nursing unit leader's role. Online Journal of Issues In Nursing, 16(3), 3. doi:10.3912/OJIN.Vol16No03Man03

Society of Human Resources Management. (2008). Leadership Competencies. Retrieved from http://www.shrm.org/research/articles/articles/pages/leadershipcompetencies.aspx

The Joint Commission. (2012). Joint Commission Center for Transforming Healthcare releases targeted solutions tool for hand-off communication. Retrieved from http://www.jointcommission.org/assets/1/6/TST_HOC_Persp_08_12.pdf

Watts, M. (2013). Growing the 'I' and the 'We' in transformational leadership: The LEAD, LEARN & GROW model. *Coaching Psychologist, 9*(2), 86-99.

Wakefeild, D.S., Ragan, R., Brandt, J., &Tregnago, M. (2012). Making the transition to nursing bedside shift reports. *The Joint Commission Journal on Quality and Patient Safety, 38*(6), 243-253.

Leadership is not about the size of your ego, it about your ability to respect the people you follow and inspire those who follow you (Newman, 2016)

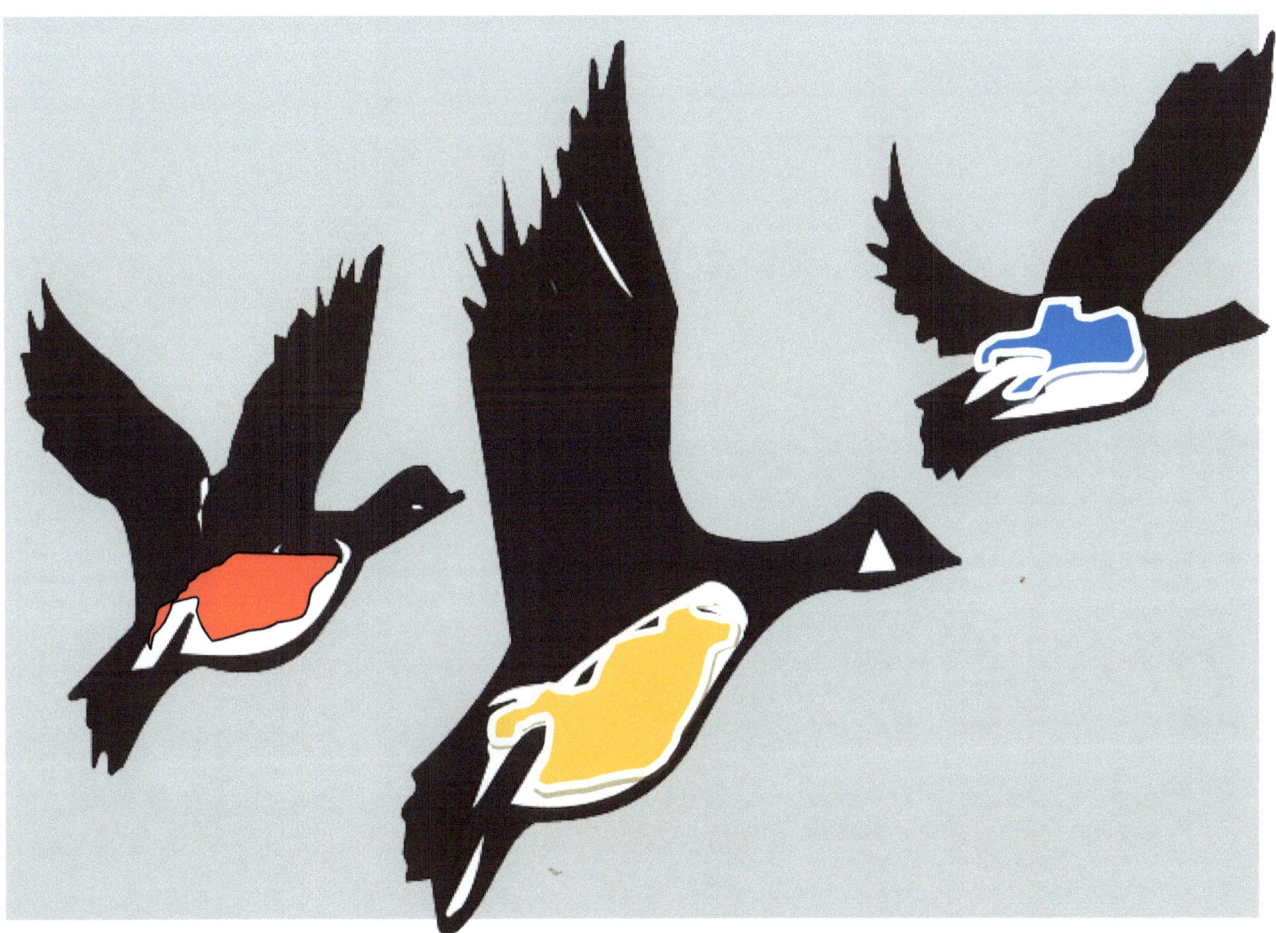

LinkedIn: https://www.linkedin.com/in/rudolph-newman-0aa49239

Tweet Me: @newman225Rudy

https://www.facebook.com/rudolph.newman.965